Sugar Free-Dom

How To Kick The Sugar Demon Out Of Your Life

John Rope

I0412324

Simple Information Publishing

This book is part of the Simple Nutrition Series covering various aspects of nutrition and weight control. They are designed on a modular basis so that key elements are included with each topic, at least in brief form, to keep the length of the book down and prevent the user having to refer to another book for explanation all the time. Obviously a book in the series covering that topic will be more informative and detailed.

Other Books in the Simple Nutrition Series by John Rope

Why Diets Don't Work (And What We Can Do About It)*

The Low Glucose-Load- Low Blood Sugar Diet*

The Psychology Of Weight Loss*

Be Your Own Diet Expert*

The Psychology Of Weight Loss*

Design Your Own Diet *

How To Start Intermittent Fasting A Simple Guide (Available soon)

A Beginners Guide to Starting A Low Carb Diet (Available soon)

Design Your Own Diet (Available soon)*

The Great Diet Conspiracy (Available soon)

* Work Book/Journal (available soon)

Published by Simple Information Publishing
© John Rope 2019

To my darling wife Barbara

Table of Contents

Introduction

Part One

Why Would You Want to Kick Out Sugar Anyway?

Introduction

Hi, my name is John Rope.

Until recently I was the Sugar Demon's servant. I did exactly what he bade me to do and increased sugar in my life, which he packaged for me in so many delightful ways, always telling me:

"Maximise sugar in your life, sugar is your only source of energy, sugar is good for you, sugar is your friend."

But I discovered this was all lies.

I stayed with the Sugar Demon only long enough to find out his tricks and his lies and then left him for good.

In this book I want to pass on to you what I learned in the hope you too can kick him out of your life.

Part One

Why Would You Want to Kick Out Sugar Anyway?

Chapter 1
A Brief History Of Sugar

Why are we so fond of sugar?
Our fondness for sugary sweet things seems to have its roots in a kind of unsigned pact between our ancestors and plants. In nature sweet things are non-poisonous and harmless while poisonous things are usually bitter or sour.

For all animal species this was an important distinction because they could trust plants to give us nutritious non-poisonous food if the food was sweet.

In the case of animals this meant the animal would eat the fruit and the seeds they contained. Once the food was digested and had passed through the animal the seed would be deposited some distance away complete with fertiliser! In this way animals helped plants propagate themselves and animals were provided with nutritious food.

As far as humans were concerned I cannot tell you if they ate the fruits and deposited the seed somewhere else but this abundance of food allowed them to put on weight before the winter because of the sugar content of the fruit, which gave them an extra insulating layer during the cold and fuel when food was very scarce.

In a nutshell: Sugar was an indicator of food safe to eat and provided much needed boost to our ancestors calories before winter.

Sugar, in the form of sugar cane, has been has been cultivated as a crop by Man for as long as there has been agriculture.

At first it was probably just chopped up and chewed but very soon, as early as 8000 years ago, mechanical means were invented to crush the sugar out of the sugarcane.

Cultivation of sugarcane slowly spread from South East Asia to the Mediterranean from where it was eventually exported to the rest of Europe.

Nevertheless it was not until the early 20th century sugar became widely available and affordable due to the increased processing of sugar beet, because of the First World War. In the 17th and 18th centuries it was called white gold and it made vast fortunes, particularly for aristocratic investors in the Caribbean Islands where they took advantage of the climate and the wide availability of slave labour to make themselves even richer.

After the Second World war another re-volution took place in sugar production when high fructose corn syrup was invented by a Japanese researcher. This sugar, is sweeter and cheaper than any other sugar and is widely used in the commercial food industry industry. It has been called Japan's revenge for losing the war.

There is so much money tied up with sugar production and all the allied food processing and manufacture which use sugar. It represents a huge part of the economies of both the developed and third world.

This has meant the development of huge pressure and lobbying power in the hands of the industries involved and an unholy alliance between certain politicians, political parties and mega business to promote and market sugar and to downplay the harm which it can do. For more details see my book 'The Great Diet Conspiracy," available on Kindle soon.

In a Nutshell: Sugar has been sought after and cultivated by man since agriculture began. Its rarity and price, up until the 20th century, made it a rich man's luxury. The rest of us were protected from its harmful effects by that fact.

Chapter 2
Our metabolism

Our metabolism is the sum total of all the chemical reactions in our bodies necessary to sustain life and it uses energy to function. Our metabolic rate is the rate we use energy to achieve all our bodily functions.

One energy source is carbohydrates. or carbs which are converted into glucose sugar in the blood stream and this 'fuel' enters the cells through the action of the hormone insulin. It is the presence of sugar in the blood stream which stimulates the release of insulin by the pancreas.

The amount of insulin released is dependent on the amount of glucose obtained from the food. Processed carbs like sugar, white bread and white rice give rise to a very rapid and high spike in blood glucose and a corresponding rise in blood insulin levels.

In a nutshell: Glucose from carbs generates an equal response from blood insulin. It is the job of insulin to keep the levels of blood glucose down.

Insulin resistance

Excess glucose in the bloodstream leads to a parallel excess of insulin production which can lead to chronic 'insulin resistance' whereby cells are unable to accept glucose as fuel, even when they need it. This leads to high blood sugar levels and high insulin levels.

When prolonged this leads to body wide inflammation which can damage the organs of the body, a condition known as the 'metabolic syndrome', a collection of diseases which tend to group together. These include overweight, heart disease, type 2 diabetes, hypertension, stroke, polycystic ovary syndrome, dementia and asthma. If you have one you are likely to have one or more of the others. This topic and others related to it are dealt with in detail in my companion book 'Be Your Own Diet Expert,' available on Kindle.

In a nutshell: If this we fail to keep blood glucose levels down then the high levels which result cause a serious disorder known as insulin resistance. This in turn causes inflammation in the body and can eventually cause damage to the organs of the body and the arteries. This is known as the metabolic syndrome.

Our metabolic rate is not a constant thing. It can vary from day to day and even from hour to hour. If we eat a meal our metabolic rate is boosted as we digest and store the nutrients from the food. This is known as the thermic effect of food.

If we eat more today than we did yesterday then our metabolic rate rises next day to compensate. If we eat less our metabolic rate will drop next day.

If we eat a great deal less in terms of calories, as in a very low calorie diet, our metabolic rate can drop like a stone to a point where we can gain weight, even on lower than normal calorie intake.

In a nutshell: In this way our bodies regulate our energy intake against our energy expenditure and energy needs. But things can go wrong.

Sugar gives us almost instant energy and high blood glucose spikes followed by high insulin spikes. This can train the pancreas to over produce insulin and lead to the familiar sugar rush followed by sugar crash as the high insulin levels clear away the glucose from our blood double quick. This leaves a lot of insulin in the system with nothing to do except cause trouble.

Recent research has shown a small amount of a sweet substance in solution (sucrose or saccharine), just held in the mouth for a few seconds and then spat out, can generate an insulin spike as the pancreas gears up for a sugar inrush. The molecules in question a too large to be absorbed into our mouth tissues and enter the blood stream. The effect is based purely on taste alone.

Our bodies are learning machines. We must teach them to anticipate the right things in what we eat if we don't want them doing things which are harmful to our health.

In a nutshell: Metabolic rates vary according to what we are eating and doing. Our bodies can learn from our activities what to expect from us and can adjust to keep our energy use and therefore our weight under control and reasonably constant. Avoiding sugar is an effective way to keep our bodies learning healthy adjustments.

Chapter 3
A Spoonful of Sugar

What sugar does

The famous line from the Mary Poppins song should read, "A spoonful of sugar makes the pounds pile on." Sugars are half way there, when it comes to converting carbs into glucose in the blood stream, causing rapid rises in blood glucose and consequent rises in blood insulin levels.

As saturated fat has been removed from the food the flavour has deteriorated and to counter this more salt has been added which can make the food too sour for most people and to counteract this, more sugar has been added.

Sugars like sucrose (table sugar) and high fructose corn syrup, end up in the blood steam as glucose and fructose.

Glucose is the packed away into the cells of the body by the action of insulin and under normal circumstances only a small fraction is converted into fat and that is recycled into fatty acids overnight which are burned as we sleep.

There is the clue to our undoing! When large amount of processed carbs like sugar are eaten, as in, cheese cake and ice cream and biscuits, weight gain and disease result.

In my companion book 'Be Your Own Diet Expert' I analyse the most popular diets and what they have in common. Some points are relevant here:

All controlled sugar and processed carbohydrates directly or indirectly.

All agree that high levels of insulin are the root cause of fat accumulation.

All emphasised whole food and avoiding commercial food because of sugar and other additives.

Permanently raised levels of insulin in the blood, cause more and more blood glucose to be turned to fat and to sugar cravings to quick fix the experienced energy deficit.

Some fructose is converted into fat by the liver and 30% goes straight into our fat stores where it is unlikely to be wholly burned in our overnight switch from burning glucose to burning fats.

Fructose is the most harmful sugar because it not only lays down fat but it also creates high amounts of VLDL ('bad') cholesterol and raises blood triglycerides which are both markers for heart disease. It affects our brain centres dealing with satiety and reward causing us to feel hungry longer and need more sugar to get the same buzz.

In short sugar is addictive.

Fructose is contained in both table sugar and high fructose corn syrup, a new form of sugar widely used by the food industry in large amounts and which makes us addicted to their foods. If the brain, together with our endocrine system, is our command and control system for regulating our weight, then excess sugar along with other refined carbs can bomb it out of existence, leaving us at the mercy of out of control weight gain.

Many soft drinks and processed foods contain high amounts of sugar to make them more palatable and the amounts of sugar we consume are often unknown to us as in restaurant food for instance.

Recently the World health Organisation has proposed to cut its recommended maximum dose of added sugar in half from 10 per cent of total calories to 5 per cent of total calories, that is about 110 calories a day or seven teaspoonfuls of sugar from all sources (all added sugar from drinks, cakes, pies etc, except naturally occurring sugars such as in fruit).

This has been widely welcomed, whether it will be enough remains to be seen.

In a nutshell: Sugars like sucrose and high fructose corn syrup contain glucose and fructose and cause inflammation and damage to our health. They raise blood sugar and insulin leading to weight gain.

Chapter 4
John Yudkin and the Sugar Giants

A man out of time

In 1972 John Yudkin, a physiologist and nutritionist, wrote a controversial book about the dangerous effects of sugar called 'Pure White and Deadly'; which faced a storm of criticism when it was published.

In a world where fat was being made the patsy for overweight and the metabolic syndrome, he was pilloried by his colleagues, despite the fact that he mobilised a wealth of information and data to support his case.

The sugar industry and the sugared drinks industry particularly, campaigned against him and he was ostracised by his peers, many of whom were in the employ or pay of the sugar giants. He had dared to challenge the big lies of the sugar industry and he suffered for it.

In this way a siren voice was silenced and what I call 'the big lies juggxrnaught' rolled on silencing anyone who cried foul.

Robert Lustig MD, Director of Weight Assessment for Teen and Child Health at the University of California, San Francisco, produced a University of California information video four years ago called "Sugar: The Bitter Truth" which gave chapter and verse on this 'poison'.

Lustig did better than Yudkin because he was not only able to put solid scientific evidence forward to back his claims, but he made them on the Internet and his webcast went viral. That remains the case to this day. The genie was out of the bottle as far as the sugar industry was concerned and we must all make sure it stays out.

One 'fact' from his lecture is worth considering here. One can of soft drink per day for a year equals 15.5 lbs. of fat per year, at least in theory.

It is worth noting the table sugar we buy from the supermarket breaks down into fifty percent fructose and fifty percent glucose, when it is digested.

Glucose is the packed away into the cells of the body by the action of insulin and under normal circumstances only a small fraction is converted into fat and that is normally recycled into fatty acids overnight which are burned as we sleep.

When we are overweight however that process all but stops and we need to reestablish it to get weight off and keep it off.

In a nutshell: Past attempts to bring out the harm sugar can do were silenced by the sugar industry, until Robert Lustig made an internet video which could not be silenced. Glucose is a source of fuel which is packed into the cells by the hormone insulin.

Fructose
The most harmful sugar is fructose. Fructose is the sugar found in nature, in fruits and vegetables. In small quantities, in this form, it is harmless because to quote Lustig "Nature packages the poison with the antidote— fibre."

Fibre comes in two forms, soluble and insoluble. The soluble form becomes gell like in contact with water and the insoluble is the stringy sort most people associate with the term. The soluble gell sticks the fibrous component to the wall of the small intestine.Together they form a barrier to the rapid absorption of sugars into the blood stream and later feed the good bacteria in the large intestine.

Unfortunately, fructose can be produced in huge quantities by the processing of maize corn (known as 'sweet corn' in the UK), and this product, high fructose corn syrup (HFCS), is used by the catering and food manufacturers as a cheap way to sweeten their products. It contains a higher proportion of fructose to glucose than table sugar and no fibre, the antidote found in fruit and vegetables. It is added to processed food in large quantities.

In an article in Nature Lustig argues the fructose is a poison, dealt with in the body by the liver (as are all poisons) where most of it is processed directly into fat and goes straight to our fat stores.

Fructose also induces resistance to the satiety hormone leptin which is released by the fat cells when we start to store fat and tells the brain we have had enough so it acts as an off switch. Fructose interferes with this by increasing triglycerides in the blood stream which reduces the transport of leptin to the brain. When that happens we don't know when we have had enough and we remain under a constant hunger drive.

A high sugar diet has the effect of increasing the sensitivity to another important endocrine messenger, ghrelin, which signals to the brain we are hungry.

This effect can be present for some time after cessation of eating excessive sugars, and is probably one of the causes of the sugar craving reported by people in the early stages of carb control.

Glucose vs Fructose

In a study comparing people drinking pure glucose drinks, and those drinking pure fructose drinks, researchers found the fructose group produced more VLDL ('bad') cholesterol and higher levels of insulin resistance than the glucose group.

Examples given by Professor Lustig

Lustig claims if you eat 120 calories of Glucose (two slices of bread), then in a well regulated individual, only 1/2 calorie is turned into VLDL-the supposed artery blocking form of cholesterol.

In 120 calories of sucrose (a glass of juice) there are 60 calories of glucose (resulting in 1/4 calorie turning into VLDL) but the 60 calories of fructose goes straight to the liver, where it is processed as a poison and produces a lot of VLDL and fat and an increase in fat droplets in the liver (leading to a fatty liver) It also induces the state insulin resistance in the cells which prevents glucose from being stored in the cells. Instead the glucose remains in the blood stream where it is an inflammatory agent, eventually causing the symptoms of type 2 diabetes.

It also interferes with the effect of the satiety hormone leptin and increases the effect of the hunger hormone grhelin so that we do not know when we have had enough and remain hungry.

A waste product of this sugar processing is uric acid. Uric acid causes gout and leads to high blood pressure.

Refined sugar is not benign, it is a poison!

In a nutshell: Fructose is a dealt with by the liver as a poison. It generates body fat, high levels of bad cholesterol, increases triglycerides. The concentration of sugars in juice, particularly sweetened juice, produces high insulin levels so the liver is stimulated to turn most of the sug-

ar into fat. This in turn produces rapid insulin resistance if repeated day after day.

Chapter 5
The Evidence Against Sugar

The Proof of the (Sweet) Pudding

However, as Lustig points out, all of this evidence is correlation not cause. Until recently the methodology to produce what is known as causal medical inference, as far as sugar is concerned, was missing.

In 2013 a team from the University of California under Lustig finally tied sugar to one of the major metabolic syndrome diseases, type 2 diabetes.

In a study of 204 countries they showed that there is a direct causal connection between sugar consumption and the incidence of type 2 diabetes, using a statistical technique borrowed from economics called econometric analysis. It is unlikely that sugar is innocent when it comes to the other metabolic syndrome diseases.

They took four major, world wide, medical and economic data bases from 204 countries and melded them together. They were able to show a direct connection between sugar consumption and type 2 diabetes.

Their data meet what is known as the Bradford-Hill criteria for causal medical inference.

They showed:

Directionality- When sugar consumption increased type 2 diabetes went up, but when sugar consumption went down, type 2 diabetes went down.

Duration- the longer the exposure the greater the incidence of type 2 diabetes.

Dose- The more sugar consumed the greater the incidence of type 2 diabetes.

Precedence- Changes in sugar consumption preceded changes in type 2 diabetes by about three years. Type 2 diabetes increases did not precede increases in sugar consumption.

Lustig and his colleagues found every extra 100 calories/person/day of table sugar increased diabetes prevalence by 0.8%.

For sugared drinks 150 extra calories increased diabetes 11 fold.

Lustig estimates 26% of diabetes in America is due solely to sugar. The remaining 73% consists of diabetes due other carbs and type 1 diabetes (5-10%).

Thus eliminating sugar, or at least bringing sugar consumption down, would have a significant on the prevalence of diabetes.

Sugar cravings and addiction can be tackled using a low carb high fat diet (See my companion volume "A Beginners Guide to The Low Carb Diets" available soon on Kindle) and or the Ten Percent program outlined below.

In a nutshell: Sugar (both table sugar and high fructose corn syrup) cause type 2 diabetes-proven. Do you want to bet that sugar doesn't cause obesity and all the other metabolic syndrome diseases to the same extent? Bet you don't.

The top 10 sugar consumers
1. U.S.A.

126.4 grams of sugar per person day.

Obesity rate 39.6%

2. Germany

102.9 grams per person per day.

Obesity rate 25%

3. Netherlands

102.5 grams per person per day.

Obesity rate 19%

4. Ireland

96.7 grams per person per day.

Obesity rate 23%

5. Australia

95.6 grams per person per day.

Obesity rate 31.0%

6. Belgium

95 grams per person per day.

Obesity rate 22.0%

7. United Kingdom

93.2 grams per person per day.

Obesity rate 28.7%

8. Mexico

92.5 grams per person per day.

Obesity rate 30.9%

9. Finland

91.5 grams per person per day.

Obesity rate 23.0%

10. Canada

89.1 grams per person per day.

Obesity rate 26.7%

In a nutshell: A quick inspection of the figures above reveals a close but not perfect link between sugar consumption and obesity and this is confirmed by more systematic data as we shall see below.

Part 2

You And Sugar

Chapter 6
Sugar Addiction

Is sugar addictive?
Some people feel a compulsion to eat sugar throughout the day, sometimes called a 'sugar rush', or more recently 'a sugar addiction'. But, is this really an addiction?

An addictive substance is one which causes a psychological and physiological dependence on it. It has the attributes of tolerance, meaning you need more of it obtain the same amount of reward and withdrawal symptoms, meaning you feel physical and emotional distress when it is unavailable.

Sugar in small doses does not do this, although it does have a marked effect on the pleasure centres of the brain. For most of us, just the thought of ingesting a sugary morsel can generate a marked sense of pleasure. When this sense of pleasure is overindulged, as it is in modern foods and candies, it triggers the same addictive processes in the pleasure centres of the brain which apply to all other addictive substances.

The effects of fructose on the brain mentioned above also have a long term effect. Over time sugars, and particularly fructose alter the reward centres of the brain causing them to become less responsive so that more and more sugar intake is needed for the same reward experience.

That is why food manufacturers add sugar to everything, including savoury foods. Addicts always want more and so they sell more. Since all carbs generate glucose sugar in the bloodstream this applies to all processed carbs.

Our old friend leptin comes into, or rather, out of play here too. Leptin attenuates the activity of the centres of the brain which determine the attractiveness of food thus doubling its 'off switch' function. When leptin is disable for any reason, this is lost and food we don't need still looks good. When combined with insulin resistance this effect is doubled.

Fact: If it says 'low fat' it means 'more sugar and salt'. Salt is used to compensate for the decrease in palatability caused by removing the fat but increased salt on its own would also be unpalatable and so sugar is added to compensate and make the food more addictive.

Advanced glycation end products, AGEs

Emerging evidence for the deadly effects of sugar involve what is known as the glycation effect. Glycation occurs when proteins and fats combine with sugar to form AGEs or Advanced Glycation End products . AGEs are part of the ageing process and speed up ageing in all parts of the body.

Glucose can also attach itself to the haemoglobin in the blood and this glycation effect is what allows doctors to estimate the amount of glucose which has present for two to three months in the bloodstream. Glycation makes blood cells stick together, eventually making them too big to travel down small capillaries which become blocked, causing areas of our bodies to die off.

This is why diabetics loose circulation in their extremities and eventually have to have toes and then feet amputated together with possibly losing their sight.

Studies have shown that excess glycation accounts for the increased mortality not only of diabetics but also the whole population.

In a nutshell: If you don't eat sugar you regain the normal control mechanisms of the brain and the body and you can't have the harmful effects of glycation.

Our sweet tooth.
One of our aims of this program must be to lose our liking for sweet things. As long as we have a desire for sugar we are not free from the sugar demon.

Sugar effects the reward areas of our brain, making sugar a drug which we seek to maintain in our blood stream. We need to retrain our brain to not to expect this by removing the drug for long enough for our brain to recover.

In this context it is often attractive to replace sugar with an artificial sweetener.

Unfortunately there is evidence that artificial sweeteners such as Aspartame actually do damage to our weight control hormones and defeat our weight loss efforts, making us even fatter.

It is better to loose your sweet tooth by reducing sweetness in our diet and eventually removing it altogether.

If you must use an artificial sweetener I would only advise using Stevia, Erythritol and Xylitol which do not seem to be detrimental to our health or weight loss efforts.

Only use enough of the sweetener of your choice to take away any sense of dryness, bitterness or sourness in your food. Try to stay just short of sweetness and then reduce your use of sweeteners. You will be amazed at how good food can taste when you have not swamped it in sugar

In a nutshell: We have to train our brains to not expect sugar in the food we eat. Sweeteners like Stevia and Erythritol can help but only as a part of a steady reduction in sweetness.

Chapter 7
Are You Sugar Addicted?

1. Do you experience cravings for sugary foods?

2. Do you go out of your way to get a supply of sweet things and keep some handy?

3. Do your cravings for sweet things occur later in the day especially late afternoon and evening?

4. Are there some sweet cakes or candies which you cannot resist, even if you have had a filling meal?

5. Do you suffer from depression?

6. Do you suffer from mood swings?

7. Do you find you react to stress more these days?

8. Do you tend to put on weight easily?

9. Do you battle to lose weight when following a diet?

10. Do you suffer with fluid retention in general?

11. If female, do you suffer from pre-menstrual tension?

12. Are you usually tired or do you suffer from fatigue?

13. Do you find it difficult to wake up in the morning?

14. Do you fall asleep in the evening or when resting during the day?

If you answered yes to questions 1 to 4, there is a good chance you are sugar dependent, a stage just before addiction. In addition if you said yes to questions 5 to 7 you are definitely sugar addicted because your dependence is now altering your behaviour. Questions 7 to 14 are indications of your addiction causing insulin resistance.

If you find you are addicted to sugar you will need to take the process of withdrawing from it very carefully. Don't be surprised if it suddenly reasserts itself in a crisis or in troubling times or in situations where your have usually eaten sugary things in the past. In that case do not become discouraged. Keep trying using the methods outlined here and you will succeed. If you continue to run into trouble may I suggest my companion book 'The Psychology Of Weight Loss,' available on Kindle.

Chapter 8
Where Is My Energy Coming From?

Fat is good for you

You may have been told you get all your energy from glucose and you might be wondering if kicking sugar is going to leave you short. This idea, which we have all being a prisoner of the many years, is reinforced by the weakness and brain fog which happens when we start running out blood glucose. Like so many addictive substances there will be some initial withdrawal effects. For some people and these will be worse than for others.

All the research and experience of people who have gone through this withdrawal phase is that it passes fairly quickly.

In 1967 a team under Professor George Cahill, from Harvard University, showed when blood glucose is unavailable for the brain the breakdown products of body fat, known as ketones, are used instead. The same is true for the rest of the body.

This means you can replace the energy from sugars and carbs by increasing the amount of fat in your diet.

The problem is, it takes the body two to three days to make the switch and during that time you will possibly feel a little under the weather but stick with it and you will come through.

You will also need to keep your carbs under control to prevent high blood sugar levels via the back door.

If you are trying to lose weight you might be better approaching this by adopting low carb diet such as a ketogenic diet or a low glucose load diet. You will still need to wean yourself off sugar and sweetness and so the methods described here can be taken as a prelude and essential first step to a low carb diet.

These topics are discussed in more detail in my books 'The Low Glucose-Load-Low Blood Sugar Diet' and 'A Beginners Guide to Starting A Low Carb Diet' available soon on Kindle.

Chapter 9
Sugar And Our Children's Health

Sugars, particularly sugary drinks are intimately involved in the increasing obesity rates in children and teenagers. Defending our children and grandchildren from the detrimental health effects of sugar is even more important than defending ourselves.

Sugar and babies

Baby milk/formula There is no added sugar in mother's milk which has some sugar in the form of lactose which is designed by nature to be good for babies.

So few women breast feed these days there is a multimillion pound business in the production of commercial alternatives. Looking around my local supermarket I found two popular brands of milk formulae with the following additives- galacto-oligosaccharides and fructo-oligosaccharides Oligo whats? You ask. Let me explain.

Galacto-oligosaccharides are sugar molecules containing glucose and bits of glucose molecules. When ingested they are broken down into- you've guessed it- glucose. So the intelligent mother looking at these might think there is no sugar in the formula but there is.

Fructo-oligosaccharides are molecules consisting of chains of fructose molecules. Theses are found naturally in onions, garlic bananas and asparagus and counterintuitively they are not broken down into fructose molecules but feed the good bacteria of the lower intestine, vital for health. As such, they are a welcome addition to baby nutrition.

This means formula milk is going to be slightly more sweet tasting than mother's milk despite these two additives being lower in sweetness than sucrose.

Follow on foods: Most follow on foods boldly proclaim "No added sugars" but they do contain carbs like corn starch , which is quickly broken down into glucose, as well as the afore mentioned Galacto-oligosaccharides.

To what extent the slight increase in sweetness of baby formula over mother's milk starts a process of sweet affinity, leading to later sugar addiction, is not being investigated but it should be. Clearly that would be a long term study, and very expensive, so I fear it will not happen.

Young children

It is no accident that sugary things are grouped around the cash-out till in supermarkets. Mother may be able to speed past the sweets or candies isle in the supermarket but she and her children may be static for several minutes at the till. That is where children can bring maximum pressure on mum to buy sweets and candies with the distinct possibility that there could be a scene if she refuses.

This is not the children's fault. They are only doing what adults do except for adults the goodies are stacked just inside the front door in tins or boxes to be scooped into the trolly without a word being spoken.

Children are also subject to targeted advertising to which they are very susceptible. For the manufacturers this is good marketing. They are teeing up the next generation of sugar addicts.

Sugar and teenagers:

Sugary drinks are the most dangerous and fattening 'food' on the planet and yet they are specifically aimed at young people and teenagers.

CocoCola, Pepsi, Gatorade and all other sugary drinks are only supposed to be drunk in moderation but they come in large, sometimes huge bottles with many 'recommended' portions. Not many adults, let alone teenagers, stop before the bottle is empty.

The industry responds by saying that it is about self control and individual responsibility but we are talking about an addictive substance here. You might as well talk of self control and individual responsibility in heroin addiction. That is patently nonsense and an abdication of responsibility by the drinks firms.

Their other response is to provide zero sugar drinks with artificial sweeteners. What they do is to perpetuate the sweet tooth of the individual for later reinstatement of a sugar habit.

In Britain and America where schools have removed drinks machines from the school, obesity rates have gone down significantly.

In a nutshell: Supermarkets, sweet, candy and drinks manufacturers are combining* (to develop a new generation of sugar addicts who will buy their products into the future until their health fails and it is too late to save them.

It is our responsibility to save them now.

*I use the word combining advisably because I cannot prove the stronger word, which I am sure you can guess

Chapter 10
The Sugar Solution

The four point system

1. Create a clear plan to follow and write a to do list for the steps you are to take with target dates for their completion. If you don't achieve a particular date don't fret. Just adjust all the following dates when you do achieve it and carry on. It could take two or even three months to kick the sugar habit but you can do it.

Don't plan to start this on the first of January, 90% of New Year's resolutions on diet changes are junk by January 7th!

The same goes for other public holidays and vacations.

Pick a start date when you have a few weeks before such times to get used to the changes in your lifestyle which giving up sugar will cause and have a clear plan about how you will handle those difficult times.

2 Root out the hidden sugars in you cupboard.

A very important step this, as you suddenly find out the amount of hidden sugar you have been consuming. Search the Internet for replacements. If you can't find one you may have to think about making you own. In this context look for low carb or ketogenic recipes.

Manufacturers hide the sugar in their foods under different names to keep you coming back and the more they put in the more we all get hooked.

Here are some names of sugar used by manufacturers

A agave syrup,

B barely malt, beet sugar, brown rice syrup, brown sugar, buttered sugar (butter cream).

C cane juice, cane juice crystal, cane sugar, caramel, carob syrup, castor sugar (superfine sugar), coconut sugar, corn sweetener, corn syrup, corn syrup solids, confectioner's sugar.

D date sugar, Demerara sugar, Dextran, dextrose, diastolic malt, diastase.

E ethyl maltol, evaporated cane juice.

F free flowing cane sugar. fructose, fruit juice, fruit juice concentrate.

G galactose, glucose, golden syrup.

H high fructose corn syrup, honey.

I icing sugar, invert sugar.

L lactose.

M maltodextrin, maltose, malt syrup, manitol, maple syrup, molases, Muscavado,

O oat syrup

P panocha, powdered sugar,

R raw sugar, rice bran syrup, rice syrup

S sorbitol, sorgum, sorgum syrup, sucrose

T treacle, tapioca syrup, turbinado sugar,

Y yellow sugar

To avoid high sugar commercial products you may have to consider home baking and cooking. If this horrifies you, you will find any number of easy recipes on the internet and you will be surprised how quickly you improve.

Internet dieting apps like My Fitness Pal or Lose It will help here.

3 Look at the sugar content of everything you buy.

Avoid anything you have rooted out in the previous step and check the sugar content of every commercial produced food you buy. Buy nothing with any added sugar. Spend a couple of hours in the supermarket, when you do not need to shop, looking at all the labels of food you normally buy.

4 Raise the level of fibre in your diet.
Fibre is vital to control the effects of sugar both those we eat and those we produce from the breakdown of carbs.

We should eat between 25 and 35 grams of fibre per day whereas in America and the UK we rarely get more than 15 grams.

It is estimated our Palaeolithic ancestors ate around 120 -130 grams of fibre per day in both its forms and these were the guys who evolved our digestive system.

Don't get carried away. If you are not used to a lot of fibre you might have some uncomfortable outcomes to eating too much too soon. Ease more fibre into your diet slowly and let your system become accustomed to it.

5 Cold Turkey i.e. dropping all sugar at one go, is not for everyone. Like a lot of step changes this one needs to planned for at a time when you are not going to be in constant contact with sugar ad advertising hype which happens constantly on T.V..

It will help if you:

1. Do your weekly shop and then go on a total sugar ban.

2. Record your favourite commercial TV programs so that you can speed through the adverts.

3. Have plenty of replacements on hand like nuts, seeds and berries to nibble when the passion for something sweet strikes.

4. Find some absorbing activities to do until the drive for sugars abates. Any-

thing from a hobby to cleaning out your newly empty cupboards.

5. As above. Never start this in the two months over the winter holiday period. The advert and shop display pressures are too great. Ideally start it a month or two before the holiday season in September or early November then you can bed into your new lifestyle and plan the holiday menus with confidence.

In a nutshell: Get ready for the battle ahead by preparing the battleground. If cold turkey does not work for you try the 10% program below.

Chapter 11
The 10% Program

Six easy steps

If you cannot face cold turkey the 10% program is for you. As a Clinical Psychologist I found a large part of my job was to help people get off prescribed tranquillisers. I found withdrawing the drugs slowly was most effective. We literally sneaked the drugs out by the back door while the body wasn't looking.

You can do the same with sugar by following the steps below.

1. Start by cutting down the amount of sugar you add to your tea or coffee, by ten percent a day. This does not have to be precise, just make sure you shake a little bit more of the sugar off the spoon, back into the sugar bowl every time you have a cup. In this way you can reduce the number of spoonful's you use, without your body realising they have gone.

2. You can stretch this to every other day if you feel you need to, but don't stop until you have eliminated the added sugar all together. Interspersing fruit teas, which are not usually sugared, is a good

way of buffering the problems associated with withdrawal. There is, of
course, always water!

3. The tendency, of people trying to quit
sugar is to turn over to sugar free drinks
which contain other sweeteners. As ex-
plained above, the problem is the sweet
tooth of the victim is maintained. You
need to break the psychological hold of
the sweetness as well as the hold of the
sugar jolt.

4. Begin diluting your drinks with water or
unsweetened carbonated water. Add
ten percent more of your chosen water
to your glass each day until you end up
with slightly flavoured, slightly sweet
water to drink. At that point change to
pure water.

5. If you eat sweets or candies, eat one or
two less each day. If you eat chocolate
bars, spread out the effects by cutting
them in half and eating them two hours
apart for two days. Then cut the bar into
quarters and eat the quarters two hours
apart for two days. Cut these reduced
portions in half again and eat those two
hours apart but stop at 6 p.m. Save any
uneaten portions for the next day.

6. Lastly reduce the number of the eighth portions you eat by one a day.

Tip: Keep a diary. Keep a record of your sugar intake, in fact everything you eat, to track your progress and introduce some reality into your assessment of your progress.

We all tend to underestimate our consumption of those things we are addicted to, alcohol, cigarettes, sugar etc. Keeping a diary helps keep us real and feel good about ourselves.

It does not have to be anything special, a small spiral bound notebook you can slip into your handbag or back pocket will do.

Just write the date on the top of each page and record your food intake particularly sugars. That includes sugars found in any manufactured food you normally buy.

Later you can use it to record your progress in other ways or to keep a note of anything you wish to remember.

Be prepared for some sort of drive to eat sugars to be present for several months. You can expect it to come in waves or as they are usually called sugar cravings.

These cravings will star with short, strong desire at first, easing off after a while followed by another wave, less intense than the first, and then another less intense still. After a time these waves will cease I and the next time they will not be as strong I promise you. Dealing with these is so important I go into them in more detail in the next chapter

In a nutshell: Cold turkey does not suit everybody but if you can stand it, it is the fastest method of kicking the sugar demon out of your life. If you find cold turkey difficult then the 10% program works just as well. Slower methods can run at your own pace. Take your time. If sugar cravings strike see the next chapter.

Chapter 12
Sugar Cravings

Sources of sugar craving
Even when we are doing well with sugar withdrawal we can still experience sugar cravings because of other influences on our biology.

Some common ones are:

Stress

Immunosuppressive drugs

Low levels of serotonin

Lack of sleep or poor sleep

Premenstrual hormonal changes

Stimulus control i.e. the sight, smell or sound of sweet packets, people chewing etc.

Stress
We are stressed all the time, whether it is because we have a high pressure job or are having to do too many things at once, a situation most people will identify with, or we are under some specific kind of stress such as the loss of a loved one or

physical injury. Whatever the reason our body reacts with the same "flight or fight" response.

As the name suggests this is most clearly understood in terms of situations where we are   under physical threat in which case our body marshals all its resources to meet the threat and first of these is the threat hormone cortisol. It is cortisol which prepares the body to meet injury or to flee from a threat. When the threat has passed the cortisol goes away.

Lower level threats evoke less cortisol but the problem is, if the threat does not go away, like a in high pressure job, neither does the cortisol. A continuing stress like this produces enough cortisol to stimulate insulin which keeps on packing sugar into the cells leading to a sugar low. Hence a craving for sugar to keep us going.

Reducing stress in you life is a complex thing but one way which has been shown to work is to become skilled in relaxation. By relaxation I don't mean collapsing by the tv with a packet of your favourite snack and a glass of Merlo, I mean very reduced level of muscle tone over the whole of the body accompanied by a feeling of peace and well being. Some people are like this most of the time but most of us are not that laid back and need to learn to relax properly.

Try the following simple exercise based on breath holding. If you are in any doubt about your ability to follow this, consult you family doctor before attempting it. Further exercises are available in my companion book 'The Psychology of Weight Loss' available on Kindle and Amazon.

In a nutshell: Stress is inevitable but if we learn to control stress through relaxation we can cope.

Breathing control.
1. Begin by adjusting your breathing to a slow gentle rhythm. To learn how to breathe for relaxation, place one hand on your breast bone and another on your diaphragm. As you breathe, slowly and evenly, try to breathe into the bottom of your lungs so the hand on your diaphragm moves and the one on your breast bone stays more or less still. Make sure you keep to a slow even rhythm. When you have experienced this, switch to breathing only into the top of your lungs so the hand

on your breastbone moves and the one on your diaphragm does not.

2. Once you know what it is like to breath into both the top and the bottom of your lungs, combine the two so that, with each slow, evenly drawn breath, you fill both the top and the bottom. You only need to do this test once and thereafter start from step 3, below, and make sure you fill your lungs in this manner.

3. Continue to breathe into the top and bottom of your lungs for a couple of minutes to settle yourself into the process.

4. When you have been breathing in this way for minute or so, take a deep breath and hold it. As you hold your breath, count slowly in your head until you feel you cannot hold your breath any longer. At that point gently exhale and take a series of three, perhaps four, deep slow breaths until you feel comfortable again and then return to the gentle slow rhythm you established at the beginning.

5. The method consists of repeating this breath holding several times a session (perhaps eighteen or twenty times). Whatever number you reached in step 4, before you felt you had to breathe out, is

your benchmark for all future cycles through this procedure.

6. When you are feeling comfortable again, you just take another breath, hold it while you count to your benchmark number and then breathe out, followed by three, or four deep slow breaths, before returning to your slow, even breathing rhythm.

7. Once you have the cycles of breath holding followed by the deep breaths working smoothly you can begin to notice what is going on in your body as you cycle through this easy procedure.

First note, as you breathe in, you can be aware of the stretching and pulling of the muscles in the chest and the inflation of the lungs.

Then, as you breathe out, notice the pleasant collapsing feelings in the chest which seem to spread out into the body as you let go of the breath up into the neck and the head, down into the arms and hands, the stomach and the legs and finally, the feet. Pleasant, relaxing feelings, spreading out from the chest and the diaphragm, like ripples on a pond; easing away tension and smoothing away those wrinkles of fear and despair.

Each time you take the three or four following breaths you will be able to experience these pleasant relaxing feelings, each one taking you deeper into a pleasant, heavy, feeling of relaxation.

8. When you have have the cyclical rhythm established, you can add a powerful verbal control mechanism to the process by adding a key word.

The word I suggest you use is the word relax; said softly in your head, very slowly, each time you breathe out like this- reeeellllaaaaxxxx.

You can do this, three or four times, each time you hold your breath and after a few sessions the word reeeellllaaaaxxxx, said softly in your head, will begin to act as a trigger for a feeling of relaxation. Don't worry about using the word relax in normal conversation, it will only have its relaxing effect when you say reeeelllllaaaaxxxx with the intention of relaxing.

In a nutshell: Relaxation is a skill anyone can learn but it takes practice.

Immunosuppressive drugs

If you have a longterm illness like Chrone's disease or an auto immune condition like lupus or myasthenia gravis you will probably be on some sort of steroid treatment and you will almost certainly experience very strong drives to consume sugar or other carbohydrates from time to time during the day. This is because this type of drug induces insulin resistance shortly after the person starts to take it.

Drugs in this group are:

Mycophenolate mofetil (Cellcept)

Cyclosporine (Neoral, Sandimmune, Gengraf)

Corticosteroids

Prednisone (Deltasone, Orasone)

Budesonide (Entocort EC)

Prednisolone

Janus kinase inhibitors

tofacitinib (Xeljanz)

Calcineurin inhibitors

cyclosporine (Neoral, Sandimmune, SangCya)

tacrolimus (Astagraf XL, Envarsus XR, Prograf)

mTOR inhibitors

sirolimus (Rapamune)

everolimus (Afinitor, Zortress)

IMDH inhibitors

azathioprine (Azasan, Imuran)

leflunomide (Arava)

mycophenolate (CellCept, Myfortic)

Biologics

abatacept (Orencia)

adalimumab (Humira)

nakinra (Kineret)

certolizumab (Cimzia)

etanercept (Enbrel)

golimumab (Simponi)

infliximab (Remicade)

ixekizumab (Taltz)

natalizumab (Tysabri)

rituximab (Rituxan)

secukinumab (Cosentyx)

tocilizumab (Actemra)

ustekinumab (Stelara)

vedolizumab (Entyvio)

Monoclonal antibodies

basiliximab (Simulect)

daclizumab (Zinbryta)

There is very little in the way of studies on this problem at present and the attitude of doctors to this is often 'better sugar addicted/fat than dead' which is a council of despair and not helpful in my opinion.

My advice would be to take this on using a low carbohydrate diet, preferably a ketogenic diet. This type of diet is the most proficient at bringing insulin resistance under control but be aware you will have to construct a lifestyle around low carb. As long as you are on this type of drug you will be under threat from the insulin resistance caused by the immunosuppressant drugs.

In a nutshell: Immunosuppressant drugs have an immediate effect on insulin resistance and therefore sugar cravings. A low carb lifestyle offers many benefits.

Sleep problems

If you sleep less than 6 hours a night or you have poor sleep, waking several times during the night, then you are losing the opportunity for your body to regulate itself and reduce things like high blood insulin levels which will promote sugar cravings next day. Also sleep is when we burn excess fat from the day before.

Worse than the above, if your partner says you snore loudly or says you seem to stop breathing during the night or you suffer from tiredness throughout the day, you may be suffering from obstructive airway disease or sleep apnoea. In which case you need to get yourself referred to a sleep clinic for assessment and treatment.

In the UK you aren't allowed to drive with sleep apnoea, it kills both people and relationships.

The treatment Involves wearing a mask into which a constant flow of low pressure air is pumped throughout the night, opening up the airways and giving you a good night's sleep. This may seem a bit radical but take it from me, you will be very glad you took action on this, as my wife I were when I was diagnosed.

In a nutshell: Sleep is essential for health and controlling sugar cravings.

Low serotonin levels
Serotonin is the happiness hormone. We need good levels of it to enjoy life and be effective. Low levels are characterised by a sad, depressed mood, low energy, negative thoughts, feeling tense and irritable, a reduced interest in sex and a craving for sugar.

Although low down on the list a craving for sugar is probably related to the tendency for low levels of serotonin to stimulate cortisol with all the attendant complications we have outlined above. The solution is the same-relaxation but also try a daylight lamp which I know are effective. See also my companion book 'The Psychology Of Weight Loss,' available on Kindle and the next chapter.

In a nutshell: Low serotonin levels mean low mood and even depression. If you suffer from these try the recommended book or seek professional help.

Premenstrual changes

Women will be only too aware of the topsy turvy world of the premenstrual time. It can generate many things from sugar cravings to strong emotion. Sugar cravings are ascribed to changes in the levels of oestrogen and progesterone in turn effecting the bodies response to insulin, but this is not much practical help.

Then there are your old friends cortisol and serotonin. There is usually a spike in cortisol and a slump in serotonin just prior to a period.

Put these three hormonal changes together and you can have a perfect storm of drives for sugar craving.

All the above are outside of the power of the individual to influence but one external source of sugar cravings is low minerals like zinc, chromium, iron and magnesium. Practical advice is to keep levels of these minerals up by eating more nutrient rich leafy greens, fish and meats. Avoid eating a lot more because your energy needs do not increase very much during a period. You need to look for energy dense rather than calorie dense foods. Supplements are less effective than whole food but a supplement of iron is probably a good idea during the menstrual phase.

Both a low carb and an intermittent fasting diets have a suppressing affect on sugar cravings and so these are an option. If you do not need to lose weight these can be used in a maintenance mode. For more information see my companion books. 'How To Start Intermittent Fasting, A Simple Guide' and 'A Beginners Guide to Starting A Low Carb Diet, Available soon on Kindle.

In a nutshell: A high nutrient diet like a low carb or high real food diet is the opposite of the high carb low nutrient diet our society promotes which breeds sugar cravings.

Stimulus control

This is where our environment, in terms of what we see, hear and smell, controls our behaviour. We are all familiar with the experiences of smelling a meal being cooked and getting a flip on the appetite pedal as we anticipate a meal to come. Unfortunately this also includes sugar. We see the displays in the supermarkets. We smell, perhaps subliminally sometimes, the sweet pudding, the mints our pocket, the candy floss at the fair. We hear the rustle of a the bag containing candies or sweets. All of these can stimulate an appetite for something sweet.

The best way to combat this at first is either to go 'cold turkey' and remove all of these stimuli from our home or use the ten percent program following the methods above.

If these fail then once again a low carb or fasting approach will help reduce the impact of these psychological difficulties. For more details on stimulus control see my companion book 'The Psychology of Weight Loss.' Available on Kindle.

In a nutshell: We either control our environment or it controls us. Be aware of the triggers for sugar cravings.

Chapter 13
Learn To Love Yourself

Don't put yourself down

People with an addiction to sugary commodities, like chocolate, tend to characterise themselves as weak willed or lacking in some way because, well, everyone else can resist sweet things right?

I hope you realise by now this is not true. If you are hooked on sugar it is because powerful forces, outside of us, have taken over the design of our environment and filled it full of sugar for profit.

As a Clinical :Psychologist dealing with the generality of mental health I came across people, all the time, for whom progress was blocked by this kind of poor self esteem.

There is a new movement abroad which has both a methodology and philosophy to help us deal with this psychological aspect of controlling our behaviour and it is called mindfulness.

The methodology is a form of meditation which helps us be more aware of ourselves and our surroundings. It helps to ground us in the here and now rather than some fantasy world where we are lesser human beings because we are hooked on sugar, or in pain or disabled and so on.

The philosophy of mindfulness is, quite simply put, to learn to be forgiving and generous to yourself. The mindfulness term is self-compassion.

Mindfulness does not change reality directly but it does change your relationship with it and, in doing so, it changes everything.

Simple mindfulness meditation/relaxation.

This takes about ten minutes and can be done on a bus, as a passenger in a car or on a supportive chair or a soft floor. But practice is needed to make it work for you in every day situations. There are also several stages which can follow this first step in mindfulness, depending on what you want to achieve.

1. Find a place where your head and limbs can be supported and allow your legs and arms to be as relaxed as possible.

2. Gently close your eyes and focus your awareness on your breath as it flows into and out of your nose or mouth, down your throat and into your lungs. Feel the expansion and subsiding of your chest and belly as you breath. Focus your attention on where the sensations are strongest. Stay in contact with each in-breath and each out-breath. Observe it without trying to alter it in any way and without expecting anything special to happen.

3. When your mind wanders, gently shepherd it back to the breath. Try not to criticise yourself. Minds wander, that is what they do. The act of realising that your mind has wandered - and the act of encouraging it to return to focus on your breath - is central to to the practice of mindfulness.

4. Your mind may eventually become calm- or it may not. If it becomes calm then this may be only short lived. Your mind may become filled with thoughts or powerful emotions such as fear, anger stress or love. These may be fleeting. Whatever happens simply try to observe

as best you can, without reacting to your experience or trying to change anything. Gently return your awareness back to the sensations of the breath again and again.

5. After a few minutes, or longer if you prefer, gently open your eyes and take in your surroundings.

Things to remember

Breath in and out from the belly.
Breath in and out through the nose.
Breath out a bit more than you breath in.

Taking things further
If you liked this sample there are several more exercises which will take you a long way towards a new outlook on life which will be beneficial in more ways than health.

One of the gurus of mindfulness is Dr Mark Williams and he has put a series mindfulness exercises on YouTube which you can access free. There are also eight week courses available for anyone who wishes to take it further.

A mindful day

By being aware of ourselves and our surroundings we can get much more out of
life We can achieve and conquer all those
things which our previous lack of awareness prevented us from doing. I often re-
commend some r all of the following to
help people extend their mindfulness session into there day.

1.Write yourself a letter detailing all the
things you are grateful for.

2. Add to the list every day by collecting
gold nuggets of your experience.

3. Write letter to your partner saying how
much you appreciate them and why.

4. Become more self compassionate:

Question all the negative self
put downs and thoughts you have

Ask:

"Is this useful?"

"Are there other explanations?"

"Are there other ways of looking
at this?" -

If you have difficulty being compassionate
towards yourself may I suggest my companion book 'The Psychology Of Weight
Loss,' available on Kindle.

5. Find a pick up-put down hobby anything from stamp collecting to drawing or
painting.

6. Learn something new every day. Try to
spend twenty minutes learning more
about something you have come across.
The internet is very good for this but don't
ignore the local library.

Endwords

Thank you for reading this book. I hope it has been of help to you. If it has then please give it a review on Amazon to help it reach other people. Thanks for that too.

Contact John Rope: john.rope@sky.com

References

Sugar Related

WHO Draft Guideline: Sugars intake for adults and children, WHO www.who.int/mediacentre/news/notes/2014/consultation-sugar./en/

"Dietary sugars intake and cardiovascular health a scientific statement from the american heart association." Circulation 120.11 (2009): 1011-1020.

Lustig R. Sugar: the Bitter Truth. Youtube video https://www.youtube.com/watch?v=dBnniua6-oM .

Lustig, Robert H., Laura A. Schmidt, and Claire D. Brindis. "Public health: The toxic truth about sugar." Nature 482.7383 (2012): 27-29.

Page, K. A., Chan, O., Arora, J., Belfort-DeAguiar, R., Dzuira, J., Roehmholdt, B., . & Sherwin, R. S. (2013). Effects of Fructose vs Glucose on Regional Cerebral Blood Flow in Brain Regions Involved With Appetite and Reward Pathways. Fructose

Consumption and Weight Gain. JAMA, 309(1), 63-70.

Taubes, Gary. "Is sugar toxic." NY Times Magazine, Apr 17 (2011).

Shapiro, A., Mu, W., Roncal, C., Cheng, K. Y., Johnson, R. J., & Scarpace, P. J. (2008). Fructose-induced leptin resistance exacerbates weight gain in response to subsequent high-fat feeding. American Journal of Physiology-Regulatory, Integrative and Comparative Physiology, 295(5), R1370-R1375.

Basu, S., Yoffe, P., Hills, N., & Lustig, R. H. (2013). The relationship of sugar to population-level diabetes prevalence: an econometric analysis of repeated cross-sectional data. PLoS One, 8(2), e57873.

Colantuoni, C., Rada, P., McCarthy, J., Patten, C., Avena, N. M., Chadeayne, A., & Hoebel, B. G. (2002). Evidence that intermittent, excessive sugar intake causes endogenous opioid dependence. Obesity Research, 10(6), 478-488.

Pelchat, Marcia L. "Of human bondage: food craving, obsession, compulsion, and addiction." Physiology & Behavior 76.3 (2002): 347-352.

Farooqi, I. Sadaf, et al. "Leptin regulates striatal regions and human eating behavior." Science 317.5843 (2007): 1355-1355.

Khaw, Kay-Tee, et al. "Glycated haemoglobin, diabetes, and mortality in men in Norfolk cohort of European Prospective Investigation of Cancer and Nutrition (EPIC-Norfolk)." Bmj 322.7277 (2001):

Shapiro, A., Mu, W., Roncal, C., Cheng, K. Y., Johnson, R. J., & Scarpace, P. J. (2008). Fructose-induced leptin resistance exacerbates weight gain in response to subsequent high-fat feeding. American Journal of Physiology-Regulatory, Integrative and Comparative Physiology, 295(5), R1370-R1375.

Basu, S., Yoffe, P., Hills, N., & Lustig, R. H. (2013). The relationship of sugar to population-level diabetes prevalence: an econometric analysis of repeated cross-sectional data. PLoS One, 8(2), e57873.

Colantuoni, C., Rada, P., McCarthy, J., Patten, C., Avena, N. M., Chadeayne, A.,

& Hoebel, B. G. (2002). Evidence that intermittent, excessive sugar intake causes endogenous opioid dependence. Obesity Research, 10(6), 478-488.

Pelchat, Marcia L. "Of human bondage: food craving, obsession, compulsion, and addiction." Physiology & Behavior 76.3 (2002): 347-352.

Farooqi, I. Sadaf, et al. "Leptin regulates striatal regions and human eating behavior." Science 317.5843 (2007): 1355-1355.

Khaw, Kay-Tee, et al. "Glycated haemoglobin, diabetes, and mortality in men in Norfolk cohort of European Prospective Investigation of Cancer and Nutrition (EPIC-Norfolk)." Bmj 322.7277 (2001): 15.

General

Overweight, Obesity, and All-Cause Mortality, Jose Viña, MD; Consuelo Borras, PhD; Mari Carmen Gomez-Cabrera, PhD JAMA. 2013;309(16):1679. doi:10.1001/jama.2013.3080

Katherine M. Flegal, PhD; Brian K. Kit, MD; Heather Orpana, PhD; Barry I.

Graubard, PhD Association of All-Cause Mortality With Overweight and Obesity Using Standard Body Mass Index Categories A Systematic Review and Meta-analysis.

Wadden, T. A., et al. "Treatment of obesity by very low calorie diet, behavior therapy, and their combination: a five-year perspective." International Journal of Obesity 13 (1988): 39-46.

Ornish D. The Spectrum: A Scientifically Proven Program to Feel Better, Live Longer, Lose Weight, and Gain Health Book

Atkins R. C. Dr Atkins New Diet Revolution: The No-hunger, Luxurious Weight Loss Plan That Really Works! Book, Vermillion 2003

The McDougall Program For Maximum Weight
Loss, McDougall J A, Plume 1995

New Atkins For a New You: The Ultimate Diet for Shedding Weight and Feeling Great, Vermillion 2010, Westman E C, Phinney S D, Volek J S.

Allen C B and Lutz W, Life Without Bread: How a Low-Carbohydrate Diet Can Save You
YouTube video "The Great Nutrition Debate". https://www.youtube.com/watch?v=feCpP40ZHql

The Zone, Sears B, pub. Thorsons 1999

Alberti, K. George MM, Paul Zimmet, and Jonathan Shaw. "The metabolic syndrome—a new worldwide definition." The Lancet 366.9491 (2005): 1059-1062.

Yaffe, Kristine, et al. "The metabolic syndrome, inflammation, and risk of cognitive decline." Jama 292.18 (2004): 2237-2242.

Rydén, Lars, et al. "Guidelines on diabetes, pre-diabetes, and cardiovascular diseases: executive summary The Task Force on Diabetes and Cardiovascular Diseases of the European Society of Cardiology (ESC) and of the European Association for the Study of Diabetes (EASD)." European heart journal 28.1 (2007): 88-136.

Fat Chance: The Hidden Truth About Sugar, Obesity and Disease. Harper Collins 2014

Popkin, Barry M., Linda S. Adair, and Shu Wen Ng. "Global nutrition transition and the pandemic of obesity in developing countries." Nutrition reviews 70.1 (2012): 3-21.

Schwartz, Michael W., and John D. Brunzell. "Regulation of body adiposity and the problem of obesity." Arteriosclerosis, thrombosis, and vascular biology 17.2 (1997): 233-238.

Bays, Harold E. ""Sick fat," metabolic disease, and arteriosclerosis." The American journal of medicine 122.1 (2009): S26-S37.

Fontaine, Kevin R., et al. "Years of life lost due to obesity." Jama 289.2 (2003): 187-193.

Bosello, O., & Zamboni, M. (2000). Visceral obesity and metabolic syndrome. Obesity reviews, 1(1), 47-56.

Chan, June M., et al. "Obesity, fat distribution, and weight gain as risk factors for clinical diabetes in men." Diabetes care 17.9 (1994): 961-969.

Fontana, Luigi, et al. "Visceral fat adipokine secretion is associated with systemic inflammation in obese humans." Diabetes 56.4 (2007): 1010-1013.

Keats, Sharon, and Steve Wiggins. "Future diets: implications for agriculture and food prices." Update (2014). Overseas Development Institute.

Calle, Eugenia E., Lauren R. Teras, and Michael J. Thun. "Obesity and mortality." New England Journal of Medicine 353.20 (2005): 2197-2199.

Adams, Kenneth F., et al. "Overweight, obesity, and mortality in a large prospective cohort of persons 50 to 71 years old." New England Journal of Medicine 355.8 (2006): 763-778.

Glossary
A

Advanced glycation end products, orAGEs

When proteins and fats combine with sugar to form larger molecules which cannot get through the small capillaries. AGEs are part of the ageing process and speed up ageing in all parts of the body.

Anabolic

Processes in the body which build tissue.

Artificial sweetener

Not all are good for you. Sweeteners like aspartame, have been associated with increased incidence if diseases like diabetes. Sweeteners listed separately here are, as far as I can determine, safe.

B

Blood sugar

Glucose.

Body mass index or BMI

A measure of how over or under weight we are. BMI=mass (in pounds)/height (in inches) squared x 703.

C

Carbs

Carbohydrate.

Catabolic

Processes in the body which break down tissue.

Cortisone

The stress hormone. A little is o.k. but a lot over a long time stimulates insulin and promotes insulin resistance.

D

Diet

What we eat. Sometimes meaning a scheme to lose weight.

Depression

Sometimes the cause sometimes the result of weight problems. Seek help! See my book 'The Psychology Of Weight Loss'. Available on Kindle.

F

Fasting

To stop eating for a period of time and then to eat high nutrient meals at the end until the next fast. For long fasts this may be a light meal to break the fast but then eating continues normally.

Fibre

Un-digestible carbohydrate which slows down ordinary carb absorption and reduces insulin spikes.

Fat phobia

Fear of eating fats, particularly animal fats because of false claims about their effects on health during the last forty years which are completely unfounded

Fructose

A sugar found in fruits which is half of table sugar and up to 60% of high fructose corn syrup use by food manufacturers. Fructose is very dangerous unless eaten as part of a whole fruit or vegetable.

G

Galacto-oligosaccharides

Glucose hidden in baby food.

Gi

Stands for glucose or glycemic index.

Glucose index

The Amount of carbohydrate in a portion of a food.

GL

Stands for glucose or glycemic load. Usually followed by a number e.g. GL10. GL 20+ is high, 11to 19 is moderate 10 or below is low. The vegetable and fruits recommended here are all GL 5 or below.

Glucose

The other half of table sugar which is used by the body for energy.

Glucose load

The amount of carbohydrate actually available to make blood glucose in a food. Some carbs are fibre.

Glycemic index

Same as glucose index.

Glycemic load

Same as glucose load.

Ghrelin

The hunger hormone produced by the stomach to tell the brain we are empty and need to eat.

H
High fructose corn syrup

A sucrose like sugar with a higher proportion of Fructose.

I

Insulin

The energy and fat storage hormone.

Insulin resistance

When the cells of the body no longer accept glucose for fuel due to prolonged exposure to high insulin levels.

Intermittent fasting

Fasting for a set period up to 24 hrs, perhaps two or three times a week.

L

Lactose

The sugar found in milk.

Low calorie diets

Long exposure leads to sharp drops in metabolic rate and slowing or reversing of weight loss.

Low fat diets

Not as effective as low carb but with enough fibre from whole food will suite some people.

M

Metabolic rate

The sum total of all the energy use of the body.

Metabolic syndrome

The name given to a group of diseases such as overweight, heart disease, stroke, polycystic ovary syndrome, dementia etc. caused by insulin resistance.

Mindfulness

A meditative technique which helps us remain in the here and now and face our problems.

Mono unsaturated fats

Vegetable fats found in nuts, seeds and olives and avocados.

Poly unsaturated fats

Essential oils such as omega 3 and 6 which are found in the ight proportions in the oil of fatty fish like salmon and herring. PUFAS are found to be protective of the metabolic diseases.

R

Relaxation

A skill which can help us deal with the stresses of life which will help our weight loss efforts. See my companion book 'The Psychology Of Weight Loss.' Available on Kindle.

S

Subcutaneous fat

Fat just under the skin. No health risk.

Stimulus control

When we are eating according to clues in the environment not because of hunger, like watching TV or just being in the kitchen or near something sweet.

Saturated fat

Stable fats which come mainly rom animals and which can safely be used for cooking because they don't change when heated to form dangerous transfats.

Stevia

Natural, zero calorie sweetener in granular or liquid form.

Sugar addiction

The tendency for sugar to develop tolerance and dependence similar to hard drugs.

T

Transfats

These rarely occur in nature but made by manufactures for margarines or by overheating vegetable oils for cooking. These interfere with our weight control hormones and can cause overweight. There is no safe level of transfats.

V

Visceral fat

Fat inside the body, surrounding our vital organs. Associated with overweight and many other metabolic syndrome illnesses.

W

Willpower

A derogatory idea often used by fat people and others to put them down. A nonsense idea. See my companion book 'The Psychology Of Weight Loss.' Available on Kindle.

Low Sugar Foods

A

Artichoke.

Asparagus.

Aubergine.

B

Bamboo shoots-tinned.

Beetroot greens.

Broccoli.

Brussels sprouts.

C

Cabbage-red, green and Savoy,

Carrots,

Cauliflower,

Celery,

Chard,

Collard greens,

Cress,

Courgette,

Cucumber.

D

Dandelion leaves.

F

Fennel.

G

Gooseberries.

Grapefruit.

Orange (not orange juice).

K

Okra.

Onions.

Kale and all leafy green vegetables.

Kiwi.

P

Peach-raw.

L

Pear raw.

Lettuce

Plums- just raw.

Loganberries,

R

M

Raspberries.

Melon.

Mushrooms-all types. Mustard greens.

S

Strawberries fresh.

W

O

Watermelon.

Meat

Other foods

Beef.

Pork.

Dairy

Lamb.

Chicken.

All cheese.

Turkey.

All cream

No processed meat

Including sour cream.

Fish

Whole milk.

All fatty fish

Yoghurt.

All without sauces

Ice cream. Home-made.

Eggs.

All white fish

No processed dairy.

Quorn

Kale.

Original sausages.

Cauliflower.

Chicken fillets.

Broccoli.

Gammon steaks.

Meat (with fat).

Nuts

Quorn

Walnuts.

Fish and seafood.

Pecan.

Butter all forms.

Macadamia.
Brazil.

Coconut oil

No cashews or pea-
nuts.

Nuts

Top 10 foods for

diets

Eggs.